Kolena -

Wishing you the very best—
Rachel

Praise for *Hope . . . Joy (and a Few Little THOUGHTS)™ for Pregnant Teens*

"Pregnancy is a blessing - at any age. For every pregnant teen, congratulations, making the decision to bring life into the world under such scrutiny is a courageous, brave, and wonderful step. Now is your time to celebrate. Here is your slice of hope."

— **Keisha Castle-Hughes,**
Oscar®-nominated Actress and Current Teen Mom

Praise for *Hope . . . Joy (and a Few Little* THOUGHTS)™ *for Pregnant Teens*

"Being a pregnant teen is very difficult. I know, I was one. There are the emotions of fear, anxiety, embarrassment to name a few that come to you during this time. You need to look within yourself. It is important for you to be steadfast, strong and positive. It is also important to have the support of loved ones. Reading this book can provide the tools and positive advice to give you the strength and encouragement to get you through this trying time. After reading the book, pick it up from time to time. It will help to keep you on the right track. Just remember after the nine month period you will have a beautiful baby that you are responsible for and you have to set a positive example for this child. Be there for that child always. He or she needs you. It is so important for you to set personal positive goals such as higher education and a career for yourself so you and your child can have a happy and fruitful life."

— **Beth Hackett,**
Mother of Rapper, Comedian, Actor, *Nick Cannon* and
Former Pregnant Teen

Praise for *Hope . . . Joy (and a Few Little* THOUGHTS)™ *for Pregnant Teens*

"A timeless message."

— **Nellie Fleener,**
Former Pregnant Teen, 1933

"A true inspiration that will help to empower many young moms."

— **Emma Gardenhire,**
Former Pregnant Teen, 1949

"This is a powerful book, that can help you improve your life."

— **Celestina Lopez,**
Former Pregnant Teen, 1951

"The message is don't stop your goals and dreams, just because you are a pregnant teen."

— **Carmen Bonilla,**
Former Pregnant Teen, 1966

"A message of hope for all the beautiful young women walking the path of teenage pregnancy."

— **Judy Brookins,**
Former Pregnant Teen, 1970

Praise for *Hope . . . Joy (and a Few Little* THOUGHTS)™ *for Pregnant Teens*

"This is a great message for pregnant teens and unwed young women. It gives pregnancy the opportunity to be the beautiful experience God intended it to be."

— **Nicole David,**
Former Pregnant Teen, 1987

"I could really relate to the thoughts, fears, and experiences described in these pages. I wish this kind of support and hope was available when I was a pregnant teen."

— **Angela Fox,**
Former Pregnant Teen, 1991

"Many pregnant teens will benefit from this message. . . I had lots of support and I am very thankful for all of it. My two kids are my life and I love watching them grow and learn!"

— **Hokulani Schwartz,**
Former Pregnant Teen, 1998

"This book filled me with strength and courage. It is a vital resource for any young mother or pregnant teen."

— **Angela Green,**
Former Pregnant Teen, 2003

Hope . . . Joy

(and a Few Little THOUGHTS)™

for

Pregnant Teens

Consciously Creating Your Legacy

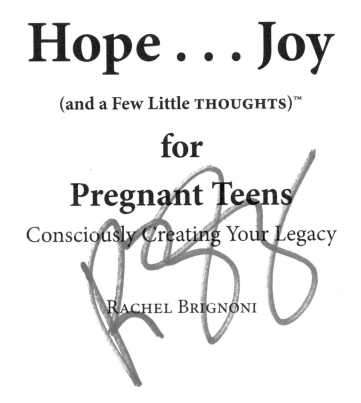

RACHEL BRIGNONI

Secret Key Publishing, LLC
Winter Park, Florida

Cover art and illustrations by Julia Menderhausen Chiaro
Author Photograph by Aimee Junnila

Published by Secret Key Publishing, LLC
5415 Lake Howell Road, Suite # 111
Winter Park, FL 32792
www.hopejoythoughts.com

ISBN# 978-0-9795626-0-0 (hc) / 978-0-9795626-1-7 (pbk)

Library of Congress Control Number: 2007905084

First Edition
Printed in the United States of America

10 9 8 7 6 5 4 3 2 1

DEDICATION

This book is dedicated to my son Kyle Gareth. You have enhanced my life more than you will ever know. I thank you.

AKNOWLEDGEMENTS

I thank the Creator, who gave me the opportunity to be a mother at such a young and receptive stage of my life; Joaquin, my husband, who loves me unconditionally and offers me a partnership beyond my imagination; my mom, who had the courage to let me choose my own destiny when I was seventeen years old and pregnant; my beautiful children for their incredible ability to love and forgive - they are worth more to me than words can attempt to express; my sister Deanna who has given me love and support throughout our lives—it would not have been the same with out her; the Berlinskys who lovingly welcomed me into their family; all my friends, especially Rachel, Kristie, Heather, Julia, Caroline, Nancy, Judith—you are the best friends anyone could have imagined. I would also like to thank the many professionals who offered me comfort, honest feedback, and practical solutions for becoming a responsible woman, particularly Bickley, Beth, Maureen, Pat, Karen, David, and, lastly, Kyle's father, for the part he played in giving me one of the greatest gifts of my life.

CONTENTS

Introduction 1

Introduction

I had a baby, Kyle Gareth, at the age of seventeen. As I look back at that time in my life, I feel grateful for the beautiful lessons that I learned. To many, becoming pregnant at such a young age was considered a big mistake. Yet, what I found during this journey was that Kyle turned out to be one of the biggest blessings in my life. Looking back, I appreciate my innocence and my unwillingness to embrace the negative opinions of others. I also appreciate the people in my life who gave me support and encouragement. Unfortunately, there were many who judged me. The change seemed abrupt and began when they looked at my youthful face and my enlarged belly. It was not the words spoken or the looks of disappointment; it was the silent shame that shot from their hearts, penetrating mine. This book is my heartfelt gift to help lighten the darkness of shame that may be cast upon those who walk the path of teenage pregnancy.

I pray I can provide a sense of understanding to those who have not been pregnant as a teenager and a reason to hope for those who will walk this path. Those who are touched by someone who becomes pregnant will experience a mixture of emotions ranging from excitement to sheer disbelief. Once everyone gets over the shock, it will be time to make some very important decisions.

I decided to have and raise my baby. However, other young women may choose to have their babies and give them up for adoption or have their babies and allow the grandparents to raise them. No matter what you choose, the decision will be difficult. Whatever your choice, I offer you support and encouragement. Any decision you make will have a lasting effect on your life. You will find purpose as you are touched and enriched by this experience. Know that you are not alone. Not everyone may bless the road that you travel, but I want you to know that you still have a huge opportunity for a successful and fulfilling life.

I was a defiant teenager, and I refused to be a statistic. The statistics would have me believe I was in a hopeless situation. I decided that I wanted to be more than just a statistic and that I had an obligation to break the stereotype. More importantly, I wanted to enjoy my life. Society's vision was narrow, pointing toward poverty, hardship, and despair. I was to believe that success was no longer a viable option. Well, looking back, it was lucky for me that this vision did not determine my future. I wanted to be successful and enjoy life. So, with a little desire, some supporters, and a few actions, I have been given a life beyond my wildest dreams. I did not fit into the typical mold of a pregnant teen, and I believe if you are reading this book you are not going to either.

You want to do more than just barely survive with a mediocre job, substandard housing, and a dirty baby. You want to live life with hope and find your inner courage as you carry your baby. You want to experience the beautiful things in life and be a part of all that it has to offer. You have hopes and dreams. You may face obstacles, challenges, and adversity, but you have a strong will. I am certain that you have a courageous heart and, most of all, an opportunity to live a life filled with joy.

I bless you and your baby. I wish you joy and a life filled with enriching challenges and opportunities as you will shine with greatness in spite of what others may believe.

Best Wishes,
Rachel Brignoni

Chapter 1

Hope Defined

H OPE is to wish for something with expectation of its fulfillment. Hope is to have confidence and trust. Once I began
to have hope, my life started to change and opportunities
were presented to me in a variety of ways. This is my wish for you.

Chapter 2

Power of Hope

I want to share a little secret that I learned as a pregnant teen. YOU get to decide what YOU want. You have the power to choose hope in any circumstance. You have been blessed with an incredible opportunity to carry a baby. In honoring this pregnancy, you still have many options. You can raise the baby, you can allow your family to raise the baby, or you can allow someone outside your family to raise the baby. It is important to remember that whatever you decide, you will determine how you feel. You are actively creating your legacy in life. Which will you choose? You can either embrace hope or cling to despair; it is your choice. Once you recognize and state your desires, the universe will align itself to fulfill your expectations. I encourage you to have high hopes for your future and the determination to fulfill your dreams. I found that all things were possible once I made the decision to accept hope into my life.

Babies are one of life's most precious gifts to women. Regardless of your age. Your perceptions of your situation, positive or negative, have the power to shape your experience. The choice is yours. By desiring to overcome obstacles and using challenges to lift your spirit, you will find that the possibilities will become limitless. As a matter of personal observation, I believe young women have resilience, perseverance, and a determination that is undeniable. These traits will be extremely valuable in developing your personal power and your character. No matter what your current perceptions, you will be required to make some important decisions. May they give you strength and guide you toward personal empowerment.

Since you are reading this book, you have either decided to have your baby or are searching for answers that will help in your decision-making process. If you feel you would like to have the baby, but are feeling pressure to have an abortion because you are being told that you're "not mature enough, you will ruin your future, or you will ruin your family's reputation," I encourage you to search for your own truth and ultimately decide what is right for you. Because of your decision, not only will you learn more over the next few weeks, months, and years, but you will also have the opportunity to become wise, loving, selfless, and honorable. You have also been given an incredible opportunity to experience hope and joy throughout this process. I believe that by carrying this baby you will become aware of your significance as well as your opportunities for abundance in life. YOU have the power to transform this experience by realizing that your attitude will make all the difference as your life changes.

Generally, having a baby as a young adult may seem like a failure or mistake, but this does not have to be the case. Do not accept negative judgment from others, and avoid self-condemnation by feeling bad or guilty. This will only attract pain and despair into your life. By avoiding the negativity and accepting your circumstances, you will begin to prepare for a life of hope and joy. Add a little faith and gratitude, and know that everything is exactly as it should be.

Your decisions and attitudes are the keys to unlocking a new-found freedom. You will have the freedom to live your life without regret or the feeling that you have been victimized by your own circumstances. How you react to your circumstances becomes far more significant than the circumstance itself. Live with determination by focusing on the positive aspects as well as your potential, and you will begin to open the doors to creating a life filled with hope and joy.

Chapter 3

In the Beginning

B y now, you may have discovered that you are a giver of life by virtue of being pregnant. The story begins with your baby's spirit looking down upon the earth. This baby could have chosen any woman in the world to carry it, but it searched and searched until it finally found someone it truly wanted. This person had to meet all of its specifications for its journey into existence. Not just any female would do; she had to be the perfect person. Well, guess what? That person was you.

You were wanted and needed for this spirit to make the transition to earth. This baby feels you are perfectly designed for carrying it into the world. It needed someone to help it develop from an invisible particle into a human being, and you were chosen. Even if no one, including you, understands why this has happened, have faith in knowing that it is for a very special purpose. The reason may or may not be clear, but trust that you are ready for this role and the baby was intended to be carried by you. Luckily for this baby, you graciously, or not so graciously, agreed to accept this life-changing event. That is precisely why you and not someone else will be having this baby. You are the female of choice, and you have agreed to allow this baby's infinite little spark of energy to develop in your womb. This is the first act of love you have given to your baby.

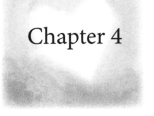

Chapter 4

Changes You Encounter

Spoken and unspoken messages will come from many different sources throughout your lifetime. Typically, these messages are intended to guide you through the complexities of life. However, depending on your circumstances, some may work to hold you back from realizing your true potential. In our culture, we send a very strong message to our youth about teen pregnancy. In an effort to decrease teen pregnancy, most campaigns stress associated poverty, hardship, and limited opportunities for success. These messages are intended to prevent teen pregnancy, but offer very little hope for those who become pregnant. The lasting effect of these messages can weaken your power, so I encourage you to disregard them immediately. It is important to realize that you are responsible for your thoughts about yourself, your situation, and your baby. It is critical to let go of disparaging thoughts and find new hope that will result in love and support. These new messages will be vital in empowering yourself.

Life will change once you become a pregnant teen. You will never again be a "normal" teenager because you will have the gift of a life growing inside you. Pregnancy will change your world view. You are now faced with making very important decisions over the next several months. These decisions will permanently affect you and your baby. You will determine your baby's destiny. This will no doubt be one of the most significant experiences of your life. I encourage you to ask family and friends for support during this time. However, you are the ultimate decision-maker. You alone will have to live with your decisions.

Many things will change, most notably your relationships with family and friends. You will no longer be seen in the same way. You will also experience physical, emotional, and mental changes, which will affect how you interact with others. Family and friends may not understand what you will experience, and as a result these relationships will change.

Your choices will forever affect your baby, your lifestyle, and your future. Like it or not, things will never be the same. Becoming pregnant and having a baby are life-altering events. As a teen, you are suddenly forced into a position of maturity. If you accept and embrace your circumstances, you can find joy. However, if you choose to ignore or deny these changes, you may experience inner conflict. Be true to yourself no matter what others may say. You may be scared, confused, uncertain, or sad, but each of these feelings will gradually lessen. Fear can be erased by faith, confusion can be clarified with information, uncertainty can become awareness, and sadness can be replaced by joy. Ultimately, pain comes from what we wish our reality to be, not from what our reality actually is.

Embrace your reality and derive power from it. Use it to create the life you want and determine your own truth. If you see your pregnancy as a mistake, it becomes a mistake. If you see it as a new beginning, it becomes a new beginning. If you see it as a personal failure, it becomes a personal failure. Your life becomes your vision. You can start changing it at any moment. Once you become aware of your thoughts and consciously choose your path, you begin the process of self-empowerment.

In the next few chapters, I will outline steps for increasing self-awareness, developing self-empowering characteristics, establishing goals, and identifying action steps needed to create a life filled with hope and joy.

Chapter 5

Knowing Your Traits

A s a pregnant teen, I realized I had no idea who I really was. I spent my life proving or disproving other's opinions of me. I had never asked myself the simple question "Who am I?"

I oftentimes found that I was uncertain when someone asked me about my personal beliefs, feelings, or character. As a result, I would simply repeat what I had heard from others. I was not looking at myself from an internal perspective. Introspection and consciously identifying some of my traits helped me realize who I was. I possessed both positive and negative traits and it was important for me to identify each if I was to improve my circumstances. I hope the following exercises will help you in this process of self-discovery.

As a pregnant teen you may doubt your maturity, decision-making abilities, and financial stability. You likely have umpteen other reasons why you may not feel ready to have this baby, but there is at least one other person besides me, who believes in you. This little person knows you are perfect for the job; otherwise, your baby would have chosen someone else to carry it into this world. I am quite certain there were a lot of options when your baby was selecting a mother. Maybe there were more mature, educated, or wealthy mommies, but there are many reasons why your baby chose you. Can you think of some of your desirable attributes? If so, make a list of them. If not, circle some from my list. If you use my list, I still encourage you to come up with some additional traits that are not listed below:

I am intriguing

I am courageous

I am disciplined

I am interesting

I am beautiful

I am respectful

I am patient

I am kindhearted

I am happy

I am creative

I am gentle

I am fun

I am lighthearted

I am loving

I am generous

I am gifted

I am athletic

I am outgoing

I am strong

I am faithful

I am artistic

I am friendly

I am smart

I am giving

I am imaginative

I am determined

I am unique

I am capable

I am inspiring

I am humble

Take a moment. Re-read the traits that you already possess. Read them again out loud. By continuing to focus on your positive qualities, you can confirm their presence in your life and help them to grow. During your pregnancy, take some time every day and remind yourself of your desirable qualities.

Now, continue to build your self-awareness by discerning your least desirable traits. This may not be easy, but it can help you realize which traits are preventing you from reaching your full potential. We all struggle with certain limiting attitudes. These can be recognized because they are the traits you wish you could change or remove. If you cannot think of your own examples, circle some from my list.

I am boring

I am selfish

I am inattentive

I am needy

I am physically abusive

I am emotionally abusive

I am pitiful

I am unimaginative

I am shallow

I am easily disappointed

I am insecure

I am punishing

I am impatient

I am dishonest

I am controlling

I am greedy

I am manipulative

I am lazy

I am angry

I am destructive

I am demanding

I am unhappy

I am judgmental   I am critical

I am disrespectful   I am negative

I am rude   I am mean

Now that you have completed this portion of the exercise, you have a better idea of the traits that block you from living a life filled with hope and joy. These are the characteristics that limit your ability to feel a sense of freedom and connection with others. Knowing which negative traits you possess will help you become aware of how you may be blocking hope from entering into your life. You may want to change these characteristics, and it may be beneficial to see a counselor to help you work on making the desired changes. With a little help and effort, you can change destructive attitudes into powerful tools for building a successful life.

This exercise involves becoming aware of both positive and negative aspects of your personality. There is no right or wrong way to complete the exercise. The benefit of creating these lists is to become more familiar with your beliefs and characteristics. This is the beginning stage of self-discovery, which will be helpful to you and your baby. Self-awareness is the critical first step in your journey to freedom from low self-esteem and guilt. You will gain insight into the reasons why you react in certain ways. Understanding your reactions will help eliminate automatic response and give you a brief moment to pause. That is the moment you will be set free. It will allow you to concretely and purposefully decide your reactions and ultimately help shape your character as you begin to derive a sense of true power. Where you may have felt powerless in the past, you will now experience power. You may not be able to change how others act; however, you can change how you react in all circumstances. Self-awareness is the key to discovering personal freedom.

Chapter 6

Enhancing Yourself

Now that you are more aware of your traits, focus primarily on the positive aspects of your personality. Keep this list of traits close by - put it in your purse, under your pillow, or on your mirror. Affirming these traits on a regular basis will allow them to grow stronger. The simple act of reading them aloud unleashes their power. Affirmation should become a daily practice. It can be done first thing in the morning, before you get out of bed, during lunch, or after dinner. The time of day does not matter as much as the practice of giving yourself positive personal messages. The more you affirm your personal qualities, the more positive energy you will create, and the easier it will be to feel a sense of hope as you get closer to creating a life filled with joy.

In order to determine my truth, I had to start believing in myself and unleashing my positive attributes so that I could bring more meaning to my circumstances. When I was feeling down, I would try to remember my positive characteristics. By focusing on these alone,

I became less concerned with others' negative opinions of my ability to succeed. Focusing on my positive traits allowed me to face challenging times with the best of attitudes.

Whether you believe a regular review of these traits will make a difference or not, the mere act of focusing on them will begin to empower you. Be patient and have faith that things will improve. Be grateful for these traits, and they will continue to nourish your hope. Once you realize you own these traits, try to add some more to your list. Try to create positive attitudes toward everything in life. A positive outlook is important for your personal growth and will also benefit your baby. Be mindful of your emotions. Try to encourage positive feelings and discourage negative emotions daily.

When you become aware of a negative emotion, relax your muscles, breathe deeply, and count to ten. If you still feel negative, repeat the exercise. Repeat the process until you no longer feel negative. Try to focus on something positive. This is a very useful exercise for combating negative emotions that rob you of self-esteem. Remember, this is an opportunity for progress. Your baby already feels that you are perfect. The better you can respond during any given situation, the better you will begin to feel as you become more aware of your opportunities for enhancement.

Chapter 7

Creating Desire

To create a life filled with joy, you must have the desire. Desire is the ignition that lights the flame of hope. As a pregnant teen, I never thought about my desires for my life or my pregnancy. I was busy balancing my fear, excitement, and disbelief. I had low self-esteem and little self-confidence, and constantly compared myself to others. I was more concerned with making sure I was doing what other pregnant women did than recognizing that my life and pregnancy were unlike anyone else's. I was always assessing my actions without stopping to determine what I really desired in life.

If you are reading this book, I believe you have the desire for greatness. On the next page you will find several statements to encourage you in finding the desire for joy. I call these the important 'I' statements, or affirmations. Repeat these statements often and out loud. This will help to bring about a change in your thoughts, allowing the seeds of hope to grow. This is an effective method of building self-esteem and understanding that positive thoughts will help to generate a positive reality.

- I am meant to live a life filled with joy.

- It is O.K. to ask questions and seek help.

- I am valuable to myself and others.

- I have many opportunities for success.

- I have the abilities needed to find my true self.

- I am no longer a victim of circumstance.

- I am going to do whatever it takes to succeed.

- I appreciate all of the good things in life.

- I am capable of accomplishing what I set my mind to.

- I have the strength needed to become better.

Chapter 8

Four 'W's That Will Change Your Life

Once you find that you are worthy and have the desire to succeed, you then need to clearly identify the four 'W's. The four 'W's are who, what, where, and when. By answering these questions, you will be expressing your desires and outlining a vision for your life.

My life changed when I began to focus my energy on who I wanted to be and what I wanted in life. I needed a lot of help to start achieving some of my goals. I was greatly helped through professional counseling, vocational rehabilitation, and weekly meetings. Participating in these activities helped to guide me on the path to success. This course of action changed my life.

Ask yourself the following questions. Who do I want to be? What do I want in life? Where do I start? When will I achieve my desires? The answers to these questions will guide you in creating a vision for your life. This is the map that will allow you to take your life in the direction you want it to go. Everything you do from the time you answer these questions will either take you away from or move you toward your dreams. The critical step is to determine what your dreams actually are. Once you have defined your dreams, you are on your way to consciously choosing your destiny and achieving personal success.

WHO DO I WANT TO BE?

WHO is defined by an individual's internal characteristics (such as patience or kindness) and external characteristics (such as a friend or nurse). This is the foundation for the type of person you would like to become. Take the opportunity to define the aspects of your personality, relationships, and activities that you would like to improve.

Now close your eyes and imagine that you could become anyone you want. Who would it be? How does she act? How does she treat others? Determine what makes her worthy. What characteristics make her desirable? Also, think of activities and jobs that you would like to do in your life. Take a few minutes and write down what traits you value most and start imagining these traits as they develop in your personality. This is the first step in identifying WHO you want to become and then growing into that person.

I would like to become _____

I would like to think _____

I would like to feel _____

I would like to treat others _____

I would like to develop _____

I would like to be more _____

I would like to respond _____

I would like to work as _____

WHAT DO I WANT IN LIFE?

WHAT is defined by the external or material possessions of an individual. What are the things you would like to own or create in life? Owning a home, getting a degree, and opening a savings account are just some examples of the second 'W'. What are the things you value and would like to have in your daily life? Use this opportunity to name your wants. Close your eyes and imagine that you could have anything you desire. Now make a list of these things.

I would like to own _____

I would like to drive _____

I would like to have _____

I would like to collect _____

I would like to save _____

I would like to earn _____

I would like to give away_____

I would like to purchase_____

I would like to establish _____

I would like to learn more about _____

I would like to become better at _____

WHERE DO I START?

WHERE is defined by the places you will need to go to get the support for becoming WHO you want to be and obtaining WHAT you want in life. Examples include support groups, churches, community centers, non-profit organizations, schools, and employers. This support is critical for change to happen. The more you surround yourself with individuals who see your potential, help you change unhealthy behavior, encourage your success, offer you support, help you identify your options, and empower you to become the person you want to be, the quicker you will see the benefits of your work. Love and support speed the process along, and they deepen your growth. You will develop faster under the gentle kindness of those who seek to offer you a hand in the time of uncertainty; they can walk with you through your journey and encourage you as you travel an unknown path. You will seek to find those who will listen patiently until you have determined a course of action to take. If you do not know the people or organizations that can help with this transition, look in the phonebook, search the Internet, or ask friends and family. Support is available if you are willing to look for it. When you are open to learning, the teacher will appear and offer you knowledge. All you have to do is be willing to receive.

We all have different needs, so this is where you start to identify your needs and locate places or groups that can assist you in filling those needs. This sets the stage for the actions that you may need to take in order to become ready to have the things you desire. Use this opportunity to find support that can help you overcome issues and enhance your abilities. How will you get the guidance you need to go where you want in this life? Take a few moments and close your eyes. Imagine that you could gain all the love and support needed to help you in this life. Where would it come from? Take a few minutes and write down the various places that encourage success or can help fill that need in you. This is the first step in identifying WHERE you can get the foundation to help you recognize your WHO and WHAT desires.

_____

_____

_____

_____

_____

_____

An example of this was when I decided that I wanted to go to college. I met someone who suggested that I go to vocational rehabilitation, which is a government program that helps individuals with disabilities obtain employment. I, of course, did not think that I qualified or that they would help me but I followed the guidance. I called the number, found the office, went to the orientation, waited in line, filled out the paperwork, took various tests and then met my counselor. He was very helpful and encouraging. He also gave me more suggestions on programs that would help pay for my college courses. I voiced my desire and then listened to the recommendations of others which helped me get there. It was critical for me to know what I wanted in order to get help to obtain those things. I also needed to be open to others suggestions and guidance. All of this combined enabled me to ultimately reach my goals.

I found hope in several different ways. I met some great people, friends who loved me and counselors who helped me. They encouraged me to become empowered. They offered me solutions, encouraged my opinions, helped me overcome my insecurities and showed me ways to become more loving toward myself and others. This support was invaluable on my journey toward joyfulness. In addition to better understanding my various traits, I also learned basic principles that helped me move forward to ensure my future success and put an end to blame and negativity. There are organizations and individuals offering support. It is just a matter of reaching out and asking for help. A support network can help you deal with the challenges of being a pregnant teen and can affect your self-esteem positively. There are resources that can help you in all areas of your life. Look for ways to build your support network. This can be critical in overcoming challenges you may face on a daily basis.

WHEN WILL I ACHIEVE MY DESIRES?

Take a few moments and close your eyes. Imagine that you could become anyone you want, obtain anything you want, and have all the support you need. What are your priorities and when will you achieve your desires? You sent a clear message into the universe by identifying your desires. You will begin to achieve these desires by using your inherent decision-making skills. Your vision will ultimately come to fruition if you are willing to make conscious choices and keep yourself open to receiving the gifts of the universe. The first two 'W's will help you determine your desires. The third 'W' will help you find resources that can assist you in building a foundation, and the fourth 'W' will help you prioritize your goals. Your goals should be divided into two categories: short-term (two years or less) and long-term (three to five years). This will help you determine the order of importance. You decide WHEN you want to reach these goals. Life is a process, and things come to us gradually. Answers come when we are ready to receive them. Preparation is needed, but the groundwork is laid when you open yourself to your potential greatness. The universe is waiting to fulfill your desires. Send a clear message and allow time for the universe to orchestrate the events that will bring you fulfillment. Your life purpose will become clearer as you verbalize your wishes. Be patient and have faith that you will receive the things you desire. Now, take the information you have written on the previous pages and put the words into categories. Be as specific as possible.

SHORT-TERM GOALS (two years or less):

For example, "I would like to get my high school diploma or quit smoking."

_____

_____

_____

_____

_____

_____

LONG-TERM GOALS (three–five years):

For example, "I would like to have a full-time job and make $25,000 a year."

_____

_____

_____

_____

_____

_____

Now that you have a better idea of what you want in life, put that information somewhere safe. This information is your vision and should be used to guide you when uncertainty strikes. For example, you have a goal of maintaining a savings account with $3,000. At the mall, you are tempted to buy a purse, but you must stop and ask yourself if buying this purse will get you closer to your goals. If the answer is yes, buy it. If the answer is no, refrain. Discipline is a necessary part of obtaining the life that you want. Short-term satisfaction will not bring long-term happiness. Hold out for what you truly want. If you take the time to find out what you really desire, you have a much greater chance of acquiring those things. Everything you do is either going to lead you toward or away from your dreams. Keep asking yourself if your decisions will bring you closer to realizing your dreams. You will become more aware of your decision-making process and the potential consequences of your decisions. Your desires may change, and so too will the answers to these questions.

You will have daily opportunities to either walk toward or away from your goals. It is entirely up to you. The more steps you take towards your goals, the faster you will accomplish them and the more joy you will feel. Remember, there is always hope. You must have hope in order to discover joy. There is no perfect path to happiness, and the decisions are yours alone. What are you going to do daily to bring yourself closer to your dreams? Ask this of yourself before making every decision. It may help you determine the outcome of your pregnancy. Ask yourself what role you want to play in this baby's life. Discover what it is you truly desire for yourself and your baby. Do not compromise. This will help you determine your legacy. For me, I had to decide if I was going to keep the baby or give it up for adoption, tell my parents or run away, continue my schooling or drop out, get married or stay single. The decisions were endless and extremely important. We all make decisions which will affect the rest of our lives. I encourage you to do it consciously.

Chapter 9

Power of THOUGHTS

I believe you have the potential for greatness, but you must decide your own life and worth. You have the power to think positively in order to rise above your circumstances. Prevent negative thinking. It may sometimes seem like you don't have control over your thoughts and that you act on them unconsciously. Remember, your thoughts emanate from your inherent beliefs. Give conscious thought to these beliefs. Particularly, if they are preventing you from living the life that you want, you must change them. If you constantly berate yourself for your mistakes, then you must change this habit. You can either allow negative thoughts to hold you back or you can transform them into positive thoughts. For example, if you think, "I am so stupid, I cannot believe I said that," you can restate it in a positive way. For example, "I am not stupid at all; it was brave of me to speak up." Try hard to avoid self-defeating thoughts. Focus your attention on the positive aspects of your character. This will take discipline and effort, but it will get easier as time passes.

I struggled with feeling angry, misunderstood and frustrated. I would tell myself, "No one really cares about me, everyone thinks I have screwed up my life, no-one understands me, and people should just leave me alone."

As a pregnant teen, I did not realize how strongly my negative thoughts influenced my behavior. Nor did I realize the importance of being mindful. By mindful, I mean recognizing what type of thoughts I allowed myself to have. I unconsciously bombarded myself on a daily basis with negativity. It was not until I became conscious of this that I had the ability to change this destructive habit. I began paying heed to my thoughts, isolating, discouraging and rejecting negative thoughts. By making room for positive thoughts, I allowed space for hope and joy to take root. I often had to seek reassurance from my support network regarding my abilities, and this support helped me to no end. We all need reassurance and you mustn't be afraid or ashamed to ask for help.

Highlight the positive aspects of life and look for the good in yourself and others. Unloving thoughts diminish your happiness and rob you of joy. Offer blessings to those around you and watch as your life becomes abundantly blessed. Focus your energy on the things that are already present in your life. The more you see the abundance you already have, the more abundance you will gain. Work on simply being grateful for what you have now. Gratitude is the key to fulfillment. Here are some thoughts for working toward a life filled with hope:

- Become aware of the good things in your life.

- Become aware of your relationships with people who care about you.

- Become aware of the positive aspects of your personality.

- Become aware of the opportunities in your life.

- Become aware of your support network.

- Become aware of the abundance in your life.

- Become aware of your deepening spiritual awareness.

- Become aware of the joy you feel in your daily activities.

- Become aware of your goals that have been reached.

- Become aware of the blessings in your life.

- Become aware of your successes.

- Become aware of your abilities.

- Become aware of the miracles in your life.

- Become aware of your gratitude for your circumstances.

- Become aware of your beautiful surroundings.

- Become aware of the limitless possibilities in your life.

Making the decision to empower yourself proves you have the courage to change your life. Now, you must do your part as a pregnant teen to create a new legacy by declaring your right to succeed. Once you have decided you want to succeed, then you must become conscious of your thoughts and be willing to take positive action to achieve your desires. It will be a conscious decision to be aware and focused daily.

I chose to raise my son. My spark of hope turned into a wonderful and challenging fifteen-year journey of love. I encourage you to discover and achieve your life's desires and help your baby do the same.

Do not compromise. Raising your baby yourself, having family or friends raise your baby, or giving your baby up for adoption are the three life-giving options available to you. Do whatever it takes to be confident in your choice. You will know in your heart that you are doing the right thing for you and your baby when you feel at peace with the decision. You have the power to choose, and I encourage you to make this critical choice and take full responsibility for it. You alone have to live with your choices.

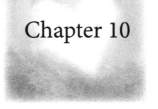

Chapter 10

Enjoying the Simple Things

I n addition to relying on supportive family and friends, I urge you to continue your search for those things that make you happy. Happiness is derived from all kinds of sources. It can be as simple as listening to music, reading a book, writing in a journal, driving with the windows down, or playing with a pet. Make the time to do whatever makes you happy. As you grow, the things you enjoy may change. Listen to your instincts. If something no longer brings you joy, stop doing it and find something else. Continue to develop your internal guide, which will help you determine what is right for you. If you find yourself enjoying something, savor it.

I have always enjoyed reading and I would turn a trip to the book-store into a personal adventure. I could not afford to purchase books, but would spend time reading titles and thumbing through pages. Once I found one that piqued my interest, I would grab it and find a place to sit. I would read and imagine I was sitting on a soft chair in my personal library which made me so happy. I would sit there until I absolutely had to leave. If the book was captivating enough, I would write down the title and page number so I could come back and pick up where I left off. This helped me avoid feeling deprived of the things I enjoyed.

Embrace the satisfying sensation that comes with enjoying an activity. This positive energy will flow throughout your body, and will affect your baby positively. Try to derive some enjoyment from everything you do.

You may not consider work an enjoyable activity; however, there are ways to make work and other things you may consider tasks more enjoyable. For example, I worked as a cashier when I was pregnant with my son. I started to compete with myself to be the friendliest person in the store. I would smile at all the customers, and always asked if they needed help finding anything, I bagged groceries carefully, and tried to show customers I wanted to help. As a result, I began to feel better about myself. I noticed that the harder I worked, the better I felt inside. If I went out of my way to help others, I felt better about myself. This can be applied to any activity, no matter what it is. Chores such as washing your car, going to school, or buying groceries can be made fun with a little effort. Since these things must be done, you should always try and find ways to enjoy them.

If you work, I recommend that you try to be the best employee possible. Be friendly and acknowledge everyone. Do your job to the best of your ability each day. This will contribute greatly to improving your self-esteem and self-worth. Trust that your employer can see your efforts. Keep your head up and know that this may be a stepping stone for some greater opportunity in the future. Work as if you own the place and success rests solely on you. Show gratitude toward both your employer and the customers. Remember that if it weren't for them, you would not have the job. You never know who needs you or whose life you may impact positively. Take your role in life seriously. You are here for a purpose, and your journey is unfolding daily. Look for ways to positively affect the lives of those around you. Good karma eventually comes back to you. Focus some of your energy on being kind and giving to others daily. The same things apply if you attend school. Try to be the best and friendliest student in the school daily. Your self-esteem and self-worth will increase. Study as though you were planning to become an expert in that particular subject. Ultimately, it is up to you to make your life a success. Thank your teachers for the job that they do. If it weren't for them, you would not have the chance to obtain an education.

Today quickly becomes tomorrow. Take time to enjoy each stage of your life. I encourage you to embrace the changes you face today by offering love to all those you come into contact with. You will give yourself the gift of peace. When you bless the road that others must travel, you will find that the road you travel also becomes blessed.

Chapter 11

Live with Joy

J oy means to be filled with happiness, pleasure, and satisfaction. As you consciously create your legacy, you will live a joyful life and begin to reap the benefits. Be responsible for passing positive messages on to others who may have little or no hope in their own lives. In time, your greatest joy will come from giving hope. The single most important way to keep hope alive in your own life is by offering hope to others. Below are some ideas for you to share your personal experiences and offer hope to others so they can begin to realize their true potential. You must seek opportunities to give a spark of hope.

- Teach others about focusing on the good things in their lives.

- Teach others about having gratitude for the people who care about them.

- Teach others about seeking opportunities.

- Teach others about developing their positive characteristics.

- Teach others about utilizing a support network.

- Teach others about understanding their purpose.

- Teach others about becoming aware of their blessings.

- Teach others about recognizing the possibilities life can offer.

Whatever your dreams, you have the ability to achieve them. You may be young, but remember you have endless opportunities to be successful and to find meaning and joy in your pregnancy. Defy the critical voice that declares you are too young to have this baby and still have a successful life. Determine your desires and make the decisions necessary to attain them.

Ultimately, you alone decide your destiny. You have the power to choose hope at any time, and build the foundation for joy. Hope allows you to discover opportunities and rise to challenges when previously things may have felt impossible. Hope allows you to believe anything is possible. Hope has the power to transform your life into one completely filled with joy. May you find hope in the words of this book. Your life story is about to change.

A Whisper of Hope

As part of your life and journey through love
There is no question that you've been given a gift from above

Hope is a whisper that inspires your soul
It calls you to action it wants you to grow
It seeks to ignite an unstoppable flame
Encouraging you to get in life's game

As part of your life and journey through love
There is no question that you've been given a gift from above

Joy is the outcome of the voice creating your life anew
You want to change and look for something courageous to do
When you have followed your heart to a new level of healing
You will begin to experience a new sensation of feeling

As part of your life and journey through love
There is no question that you've been given a gift from above

Your thoughts are lifted from the depth of your pain
They awaken your life which can never be the same
You are conscious of the doubt that highlights your shame
But is replaced ever so slowly and calls you by name

As part of your life and journey through love
There is no question that you've been given a gift from above

Rachel Brignoni

ABOUT THE AUTHOR

Rachel Brignoni became pregnant at the age of seventeen – a circumstance considered tragic in the eyes of society. In high school she was a cheerleader, honor-roll student, and a homecoming princess; life was great until she unexpectedly became pregnant. She got married within two weeks of discovering the news, got pregnant again within four months of giving birth, had a miscarriage, and eventually divorced. Facing a life of poverty, addictions, and despair, she made a conscious decision to take responsibility and change the outcome of her life. Feeling broken at times but unwilling to give up, she withstood the harsh judgment of others. She would not accept their sentiments of shame or hopelessness for her future. During this journey she realized her son was one of her greatest gifts and would teach her the value of her circumstances. Determined to create a legacy of success, she overcame many obstacles while raising her son as a single mom. After ten years of struggling to balance motherhood, work, and education, she earned her Bachelor of Arts Degree in Sociology from the University of Central Florida.

She is currently a Human Resources Executive at a Fortune 100 company where she provides counsel on organizational effectiveness and employee-related issues. She is also Vice President of her own company that revitalizes impoverished homes in an effort to provide quality housing within communities. As a Certified Life Strategies Coach her book *Hope . . . Joy (and a Few Little THOUGHTS)™ for Pregnant Teens* is the first in a series of books dedicated to inspiring parents and young adults to consciously create a life filled with hope and joy. Now thirty-three, Rachel lives in Florida with her husband and three children.

(and a Few Little THOUGHTS)™

(and a Few Little THOUGHTS)™

_____

_____

_____

_____

_____

_____

_____

(and a Few Little THOUGHTS)™

(and a Few Little THOUGHTS)™

_____

_____

_____

_____

_____

_____

_____

_____

(and a Few Little THOUGHTS)™

_____

_____

_____

_____

_____

_____

_____

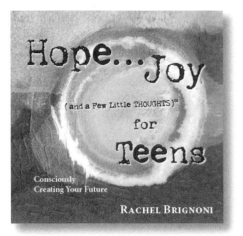

Future Release

Hope . . . Joy
(and a Few Little THOUGHTS)™
for Teens
Consciously Creating Your Future

RACHEL BRIGNONI

6 x 6 Hardcover w / Bonus CD $19.95
Paperback, $12.95

ISBN #: 978-0-9795626-2-4(hc)
ISBN #: 978-0-9795626-3-1(pbk)

Creative, energetic, and fearless, teens are moving at a fast pace toward adulthood. Faced with many options, teens are frequently at risk of making unconscious decisions that can have a lasting effect on their future. To become aware of their true desires and personal potential, this book outlines steps for increasing self-awareness, developing self-empowering characteristics, establishing goals, and identifying action steps needed to consciously create their future by realizing the power of each thought.

For more information visit our website at:
www.hopejoythoughts.com or e-mail us at secretkey@hopejoythoughts.com